Cancer
My Little Green Book

Three key lifestyle changes enabled
me to transform my health and
control cancer

IÑAKI LEGORBURU

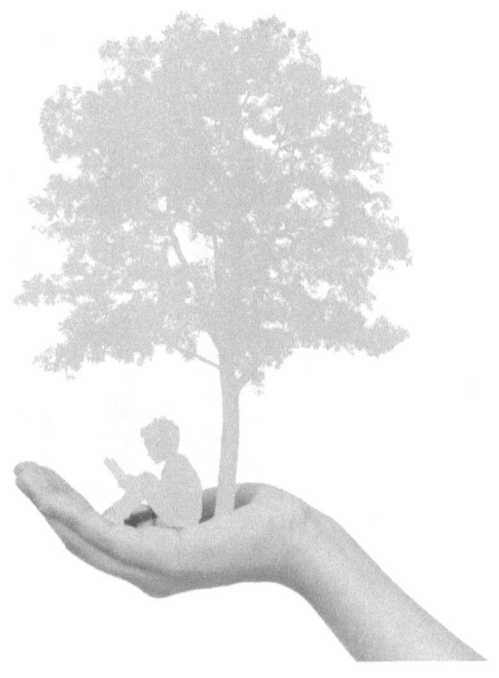

DEDICATION

To all my family and friends who found the courage to overcome their fears and support my lifestyle strategy to take control over cancer. And to Dr. Cornelis Moerman for finding the courage to pursue his pioneering work into cancer therapy whilst facing a lifetime of abuse from the medical establishment. Had I not come across *his* little green book from 1978, then I would probably not be sharing this story with you today.

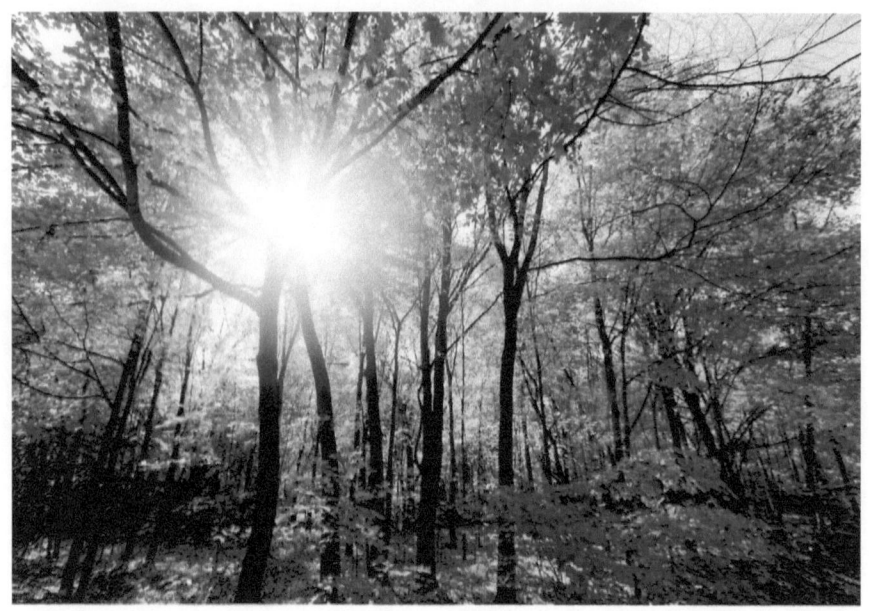

"Cancer can be both prevented as well as controlled by adopting three key lifestyle changes: a liver-friendly food plan, early to bed and early to rise, and early morning country walks. This approach is designed to revitalize and re-balance the body, mind and spirit. The rest kind of takes care of itself."

CONTENTS

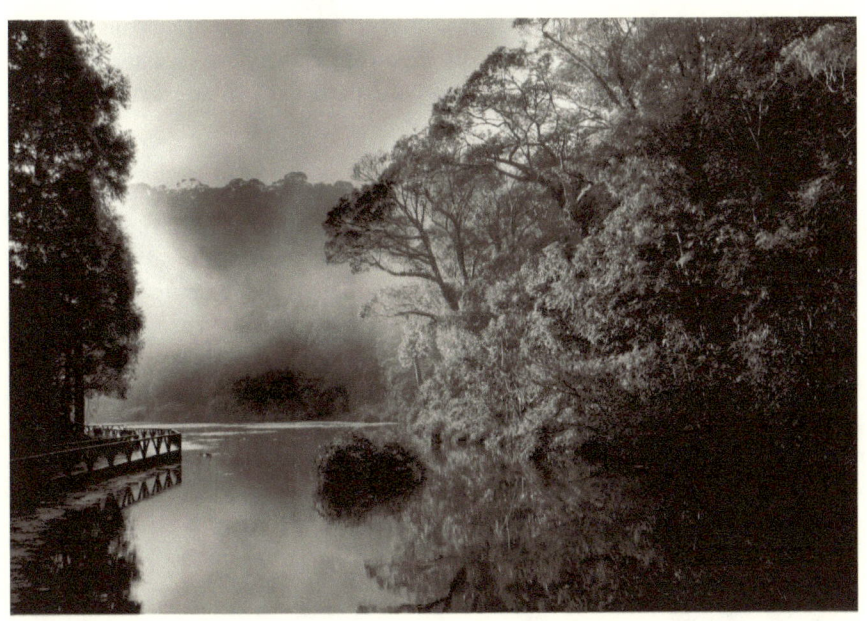

FOREWORD

"You have cancer!"

"You have cancer!" Hearing these words, spoken to me by my oncologist, triggered a long needed change in lifestyle: good food, gentle exercise and plenty of rest. Although I agreed to initial surgery, I said no to all the subsequent proposals for re-surgery and chemo therapies.

In the days that followed the initial surgery, I started investigating what had been written by medical specialists and professionals about treatments for cancer. On hindsight I realize how fortunate I was in the beginning to get hold of a 2nd hand copy of Dr. Moerman's original "little green book". Published in 1978, this book was now out of print. His writing struck a chord inside me, when it dawned on me that his focus of attention was not "foods that help fight cancer" but "foods that help restore a healthy body."

Dr. Cornelis Moerman adopted a broader approach, by exploring what the body required in the way of nutrition to become healthy again and to retain its health. Essential steps on the path to restoring a working balance between mind, body and spirit. The hard path back after many years of taking the easy path forward.

Yoga was formulated hundreds of years ago by learned men, who wanted to bring about a perfect balance of body, mind and spirit. A mixture of physical and mental exercises, breathing techniques, dietary guidelines and more. Even yoga has suffered (some would argue benefited) from our need to analyze and understand and develop an evidence-base. How many different yoga teaching systems exist today? How many alternative systems exists that share the same underlying goal of striving for a perfect balance of body, mind and spirit. The underlying universal truth is that our health can be maximized by restoring and maintaining the balance between body, mind and spirit. Perfect balance leads to maximized health. But we are far from perfect, and our working and living environments are far from perfect. Each day people, places and things affect our lives, as we in return affect them.

I came across many different and alternative approaches, that also appeared to work in practice. The grape juice therapy from Anna Brandt, the Gerson Therapy, the Medical Testament, Foods That Fight Cancer, Yoga techniques and Chi-lel exercises, Chi walking techniques, Wim Hof breathing exercises... to name just a few. Each, in their own way, has a successful track record behind them. They also share something else with Dr. Moerman's approach: they do not (yet) lend themselves to randomized clinical trails, and therefore cannot provide a scientific evidence base to support their claims.

Dr. Moerman's food plan may differ in detail from other food plans and therapies that have left a trail of success cases behind them, but they all share some important characteristics. The effective food plans ensure that the body obtains and absorbs the nutrition essential to restoring and maintaining a healthy body, and they strive to do this for a minimum of effort from the body. This is a good starting point for the cancer patient who is motivated to evaluate his/her current food plan. All to often we discover (as I did) that certain nutrients are missing in our choice of foods. I was shocked at all the processed foods, and the resulting high amounts of salt and sugar and saturated fats, that I was forcing into my body. No wonder my major organs were being overloaded and no longer able to function properly in a clogged up environment. The small clinical symptoms that started to appear more and more frequently in the years leading up to my cancer were, on hindsight, clear early warning signals. They were out in the open for many years before a medical scan or blood test could have picked up on cancer.

Although I am not following their recommended medical protocol for treating my cancer, the AVL (Antoni van Leeuwenhoek) cancer center in Amsterdam still welcomes me every 6 months for a thorough check-up to see if cancer has returned. I know that should these tests come out positive some day, that they will only serve as confirmation of something that I already knew or suspected based on my own observations regarding my adherence to the structure of my adopted lifestyle, my own sense of vitality and energy physical-mental-emotional, and last but not least, signs of returning clinical symptoms. Plenty of opportunity, armed with the knowledge and experience I have now, to prevent cancer from returning in the future.

What I have learned from my encounter with cancer, is that when I am eating well, exercising regularly and getting sufficient sleep, then my outlook on life is much brighter, I am more socially aware of my interaction with my environment, and I am dealing with more inspiration and ideas on a daily basis. Unexpected issues and confrontations have much happier endings.

Should my positive attitude and the decisions and actions that I take result in a successful fight against cancer, then that will be my good fortune. I will have been lucky. There are many cancer patients, including some of my family members and friends over recent years, who have reached inside themselves and overcome their fears with an unbelievable amount of positive attitude and willpower, and a fighting spirit that has enabled them to survive battle after battle... to their last breath when they finally succumbed to cancer. There are no guarantees in life. But hearing the words from the oncologist proved to be a defining moment in my life, during which a voice deep inside me calmly whispered "I choose life." I could take responsibility for my personal actions, decide what was best for me, and I chose life. This choice was for much more than just quality of life.

My cancer is a messenger, yet my real battles will not be against cancer. My real battles will be to rediscover myself and open up to family, friends and the universes that embrace me.

This book is the result of my journey back to life. My insights, thoughts, moods and emotions fluctuated along the way. My wording in the past reflected my feelings of anger, frustration, surprise, faith, hope, compassion and love in the past. I have tried to restructure my story into a logical whole.

At times I will repeat my words and repeat some of the lessons I have learned along the way. Some words and lessons are worth repeating, for fear that they may pass unread and unheard.

This is my personal journey, my personal logbook of life with cancer.

My personal experience? Six weeks after my operation my vitality had returned and there were no lingering traces of cancer to be found in my body.

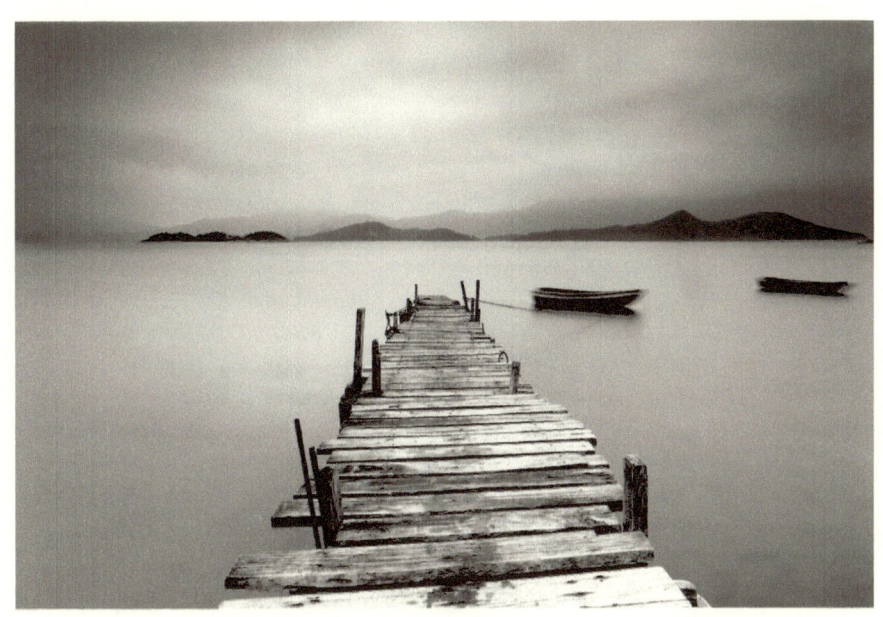

1 EARLY WARNING SIGNALS

Extracts from my diary

For the first couple of years I kept a diary for myself.

When re-reading my letters to family and friends, I find it encouraging to see that phrases such as "the vitality is back again", "improvements in physical and mental health", "changed eating pattern, regular outdoor exercise" and "fully functioning immune system" were already sowing their seeds back then, and continue to flourish today in my adopted lifestyle.

I have selected extracts from these letters to provide you, the reader, with an insight into my way of thinking and frame of mind during those first weeks of living with the knowledge that I had cancer. These insights have stood their ground amazingly well and are therefore well worth sharing here.

"The past few weeks have seen significant improvements in my physical and mental health. I love the Moerman food plan, and I am in contact with my body again. And the morning walk in the woods is beneficial in many ways.

The realization that I had cancer came as a shock, yet instead of triggering fear it triggered an awakening. Instead of a fear for cancer, my focus was an awareness of my desire to enjoy my life with my family and friends. Also a realization that the past 10 years have been a downward spiral health wise with a long trail of incidents e.g. Meniere, lung embolism, recurring erysipelas and antibiotics, wounds that do not want to heal quickly, unable to walk without crutch support this past year. In short my immune system has been steadily breaking down. So when cancer was discovered, I was convinced that the extent of cancer could well have reached or was beginning to appear in other areas such as kidneys, liver and stomach. This conviction was a reflection of what my oncologist was thinking. With my excess body weight I am in fact surprised that diabetes has not arisen yet. So I hope that you understand why my focus has not been on the cancer but, on rebuilding my health and immune system. I am convinced that a fully functioning immune system, assisted by some extra triggers, is capable of sending cancer into regression.

Did I/do I have any fears? Yes. The fear that operations, chemo treatments and radiation treatments further weaken my immune system to the point that there is no resistance to cancer appearing and /or developing further in places such as the kidneys, liver and stomach.

At the moment I am probably fitter than I have been for a number of years. Changed eating pattern, regular outdoor exercise and a conviction that I will regain my good health and that the cancer will in due course take a back-door exit."

If cancer had not appeared on the scene, then it would not have been long before the lung embolism that I suffered in 2004 would have been followed by other ailments. For the past year I have had difficulty walking without the support of a crutch, obesity and diabetes were lurking in the shadows, all signs of a deteriorating immune system. Anyway, these symptoms and others have disappeared over the past couple of weeks through a well thought out food plan and exercise and a dose of positive thinking. The vitality is back again.

I have a lot of options and alternatives in front of me, and many more questions that I hope to get answered over the next two weeks.

My convictions? That Dr. Cornelis Moerman achieved a beneficial synergy between the nutritional elements in his food plan. That vitamin C plays an important role both as a trigger to the immune system as well as facilitating synergy between desirable processes in the human body. And that it will take more than just a good food plan to get through the coming years.

I reflect on that day, that moment, when my urologist informed me 'You have an aggressive form of cancer. Why did you wait so long?' and an operation was planned in for the following week. Not much time to let the news sink in or work out a course of action for myself. I do recall experiencing that moment as a defining moment, not dominated by surfacing fears, but by an inner voice saying 'I choose life' and the ensuing sense of liberation and conviction that cancer had saved my life. I did not and still to this day do not view cancer as an enemy to fight.

As you will probably know by now, I chose a different path than the established medical protocol for treating my cancer. No toxic therapies. I focused on nutrition, exercise and sleep. My vitality is back, and judging from the disappearance of all my other ailments (joint pains, recurring erysipelas, slow healing wounds, bleeding gums, leg, ankle and foot edema, excess body weight) my immune system has been restored to a healthy state. The AVL cancer center in Amsterdam respected my choice and was prepared to check my condition every 3 months. My last check up showed no more signs of cancer. We will continue the check ups over the coming years. So far so good."

Absorb what is useful and discard what is useless

Friends and family occasionally experience difficulty following me in my actions and decisions. It seems as if I am saying one thing one day and something else the next. There is some truth in that, but it comes from my somewhat simple approach to learning and hopefully progressing, and a recognition that we are all individuals and each of us is responsible for finding what works for him/her. My simple approach is:

- absorb what is useful
- discard what is useless
- add a few ingredients of my own

I experienced my recovery from cancer as a process with two essential parts, detox/cleansing and nourishment, i.e. restoring my body's abilities to discard what is useless and absorb what is useful. These abilities got screwed up / impaired by my bad eating habits, bad exercise habits, bad working habits and bad sleeping habits, and the imbalance that resulted between all of them led me on a downward health spiral path.

Most probably I have been blessed with what is generally termed a strong constitution, that enabled me to endure a lot before suffering the consequences at a more advanced age. Had I been born with a weaker or frailer constitution, or genetic weakness, then the consequences may well have appeared much earlier. Had there been evidence of a more distinct inherent genetic weakness, then I would (on hindsight) found the wisdom to place even more emphasis on good lifestyle habits such as the Moerman food plan, daily morning walks in the forest and early to bed and early to rise. When a chronic disease is the (assumed) result of a genetic flaw, then it makes even more sense to me to adopt a well thought out food plan, exercise routine and sleep schedule.

Our bodies are amazing

Given the opportunity our bodies will recover from the worst of situations.

What does our body do when we find ourselves in cold outdoor temperatures? It cuts off the flow of blood and oxygen to our extremities, to ensure that our vital organs continue to function for as long as possible. This is a survival mechanism.

What does our body do when we experience a sudden traumatic event? It switches into shock-mode thereby ensuring that for the initial minutes we are not paralyzed by pain, giving us the opportunity to apply some first-aid to the situation. This is a survival mechanism.

In the first case we can feel the cold, which is an early warning signal. In the second case there is no early warning.

When we train physically, as is the case with running or cycling, we can wake up the next morning feeling stiff. This is an early warning that we should warm our muscles up slowly before proceeding to train again, otherwise a muscle or joint injury may follow.

If we train intensely day after day, we can reach a point where we start to feel lethargic about our training, that sense of vitality and eagerness can start to fade away. This is an early warning that we are overdoing our training, that our body is not being given the opportunity to rest and recover from the previous training. When we do not heed this warning, then it is not unusual to experience a downturn in our performance, such as reduced speeds and shorter endurance, or increased susceptibility to injury.

Athletes who get to bed late or don't get enough sleep will see this shortage of sleep impact directly on their performances. The lowered performance is an early warning signal.

When we eat too much at a meal, or eat the foods that don't agree with us, we can experience a bloated feeling, and a lack of energy to do anything that exerts us physically after the meal. Not surprising, because our bodies are working hard to digest the meal. The bloated feeling and the lack of energy – both are early warning signals.

When our food does not contain all the essential nutrients our bodies require, we see tell-tale signs, early warning signals. Dr. Moerman labeled these the "small clinical symptoms" of nutritional deficiencies. But it can also be that our food does contain all the essential nutrients, yet our bodies are not able to absorb them all due to malfunctioning organs or blocked flow channels, food allergies or certain food intolerance, or simply being stressed out emotionally. There is a whole myriad of cause-effect relationships that make themselves visible in the form of symptoms (= early warning signals) such as waking up tired each morning, more susceptibility to colds and fevers, infections and wounds that will not heal, coughing that just will not go away no matter how many antibiotics we take.

There are many of these early warning signals that are lifestyle related, i.e. food, exercise and sleep related. To name just a few more:

- skin that develops dry patches with a tendency to harden and crack as it loses elasticity; callused foot soles, corn-edged skin pores, discolored facial skin;
- chapped mouth corners; aberration of the mucous membrane; red spots and scale-like formation on skin around nostrils; tongue and inside of lips adopt a very red color;
- finger nails are hard, brittle with stripy structure;
- hair loses its shine and adopts a lifeless look;
- gums bleed easily;
- bruising from the slightest impact;
- slow healing of wounds;
- fatigue without due reason; we feel tired just at the idea of starting on the next task, even the idea of getting out of bed;
- pale complexion;
- nervous, on edge; tendency to sweat easily;

- painful joints: knees, wrists, elbows, hips.

These early warning signals can be viewed as signs of nutrient deficiency, and I started down the path of discovering which vitamin or mineral I should be supplementing. But I soon realized that I did not want you, the reader, to move down the path of supplementation. *This is the easy path forward, which is also the hard path back.* When we take two aspirins for our headache, or antibiotics for our lung infection, or supplements for our nutritional deficiencies, which is understandable given the hectic lives many of us lead, we are taking the easy path forward. I should know, I was doing it for at least 40 years of my life. The hard path back is the one in which we re-balance our lifestyle, and make some key changes to our food plan, exercise routine and sleeping schedule. When we do this we no longer need to worry about specific nutrient shortages. Our balanced food plan takes everything into account in a natural and gentle way.

At this point I realize that it may well be useful to include some information about the nutritional side of different foods and how they relate to the small clinical symptoms. I emphasize "may be useful" because I consider this knowledge optional. Much of the knowledge I acquired after I had regained my good health and recovered from cancer. I even went as far as to study and qualify as a certified nutritionist.

There is such a high degree of overlap and intertwining between the nutrients listed and the associated deficiency symptoms, that I experienced (and I still do) the information as confusing and potentially misleading if interpreted wrongly.

I adopted a balanced food plan using the guidelines set out by Dr. Moerman, and I was fortunate enough that my deficiency symptoms disappeared within days and weeks. My search for a deeper understand of why this food plan worked for me has led to the following information.

Foods, nutrients and (small) clinical symptoms

Dr. Cornelis Moerman (1893-1988) identified the following 8 nutrients that were essential to restoring the balance in a healthy body and immune system, and should therefore be present in our daily food:

- vitamin A
- yeast (we now refer to this as the whole complex of vitamin B)

- vitamin C
- vitamin E
- citric acid
- iron
- iodine
- sulfur

The list I put together for myself goes beyond the 8 essential nutrients listed above. It includes the whole B-vitamin complex and an extensive mineral list that represents my knowledge anno 2012. The extensive list did satisfy me on one important account. The range of foods in my food plan, that covered the 8 essential nutrients, also covered the additional vitamins and minerals listed. Once I established that for myself, I let go of all the individual nutrients and their related deficiency symptoms, and just focused on sticking to a balanced food plan.

I noticed how certain deficiency symptoms can be attributed to more than one nutrient, and that interrelationships can exist between so-called essential and non-essential nutrients. Even non-essential nutrients, when a deficiency exists, can apparently become essential for restoring good health. The best safeguard I know to prevent nutrient deficiency is introducing variety to a balanced food plan. There are still many micro-nutrients that we either still have to discover or we still have to learn about their role in our body processes, and there is much about synergy between nutrients that is beyond the scope of our scientific evidence-based research. Therefore my basic food plan is designed to cover the eight essential nutrients identified by Dr. Moerman, as well as the more extensive list of "non-essential" nutrients. And I add a pinch of variety to my food plan to cover all the micro-nutrients that I am not yet aware of.

Vitamin A (retinol)
Foods: Dairy products (milk, butter, cheese, cream), liver, cod liver oil, herring, halibut, liver sausage, kidney, eggs, leafy dark green vegetables (endive, spinach, kale, broccoli), carrots, tomatoes, apricots, beet, parsley, sweet potatoes, apples, mango, watercress, cantaloupe, palm oil.
Processes: Growth & repair of body tissues [resist infections], bone & tooth formation, night vision
Deficiency symptoms: Night blindness, dry, scaly skin, loss of smell & appetite, tooth decay, fatigue, susceptibility to infection

Here follows the B-vitamin complex:

Ameruïne of thiamine (B1 – regarded as an essential B-vitamin)

Foods: Yeast, sunflower seeds, nuts, whole grain products, molasses, leguminous fruit, pork (ham, bacon, liver), eggs, milk, rice, pine nuts, soy milk, sesame seed, buckwheat, whole wheat pasta, lima beans.

Processes: Carbohydrate metabolism, appetite maintenance, nerve function, growth & muscle tone

Deficiency symptoms: Beriberi, heart irregularity, nerve disorders, fatigue, loss of appetite, forgetfulness

Riboflavine (B2 – regarded as an essential B-vitamin)

Foods: Yeast, whole grain cereals, legumes, organ meats (liver, kidney, lung), vegetables, bean sprouts,, eggs, cheese, milk, fish (salmon / sardines canned), meat, almonds, mushrooms, eggs, soy beans, parsley, cashew nuts, rice, lentils, molasses, linseed, sesame, sunflower, broccoli, avocado, asparagus.

Processes: Fat, carbohydrate, & protein metabolism, cell respiration, antibody & red blood cell formation

Deficiency symptoms: Eye problems, cracks in corners of mouth, digestive disturbances

Niacin (B3 – regarded as an essential B-vitamin)

Foods: Yeast, (organ) meat, eggs, milk, legumes, nuts, salmon, tuna, chicken, halibut, beef, peanuts, whole grain cereals, fish (white), beef, lamb and veal, tomato, mushrooms, brown rice, sesame seeds, sunflower seeds, whole wheat pasta, peach (dried).

Processes: Fat, carbohydrate, & protein metabolism, health of skin, tongue, & digestive system, blood circulation

Deficiency symptoms: Fatigue, indigestion, irritability, loss of appetite, skin disorders

Pantothenic Acid (B5 – regarded as an essential B-vitamin)

Foods: Organ meats (especially liver), whole grain products, yeast, milk, egg yolk, nuts, royal jelly, mushrooms, beans, soybeans, broccoli, molasses, peanuts , beef, salmon, green vegetables, legumes, avocado.

Processes: Converts nutrients into energy, formation of some fats, vitamin utilization

Deficiency symptoms: Vomiting, stomach stress, restlessness, infections, muscle cramps

Pyridoxine (B6 – regarded as an essential B-vitamin)
Foods: Yeast, sunflower seeds, nuts, whole grain cereals, fish, meat, assorted vegetables, chicken, liver, kidney, walnuts, salmon, trout, tuna, halibut, lentils, lima beans (dried), soy beans, brown rice, hazelnuts, bananas, avocados, chestnuts, spinach, sweet red peppers, potatoes, sardines, sprouts, sweet potatoes, cauliflower, popcorn, red cabbage, leek, egg yolk, molasses.

Processes: Fat, carbohydrate, & protein metabolism, antibody formation, nerve function

Deficiency symptoms: Nervousness, dermatitis, blood disorders, muscular weakness, insulin sensitivity, anemia

Inositol (B8 – regarded as an essential B-vitamin)
Foods: Yeast, lecithin, whole grain products, oats, nuts, milk, molasses, asparagus, citrus fruits, pork, liver.

Processes & Deficiency symptoms: Deficiency is rare as the body manufactures inositol, and it is present in a wide variety of foods. However, deficiency can result e.g. from long term use of antibiotics or regular consumption of more than 2 cups of coffee daily.

Para-aminobenzoic acid (B10 – not regarded as an essential B-vitamin)
Foods: Yeast, whole grain products, milk, eggs, yogurt, molasses, liver, green leafy vegetables.

Processes & Deficiency symptoms: not regarded as an essential nutrient

Folic Acid (B11 – regarded as an essential nutrient)
Foods: Liver, hard boiled eggs, oyster, salmon, milk, wholemeal bread, yeast, legumes, alfalfa, spinach, endive, asparagus, canned tomatoes, chicken, lettuce, green vegetables, fresh orange juice, nuts.

Processes: Red blood cell formation, protein metabolism, growth & cell division

Deficiency symptoms: Anemia, gastrointestinal problems, poor growth

Cobalamin (B12 – regarded as an essential B-vitamin)
Foods: Liver, kidney, lean meat, chicken, fish, shellfish, cottage cheese, milk, eggs, cheese.

Processes: Fat, carbohydrate, & protein metabolism, maintains nerve function, blood cell formation

Deficiency symptoms: Pernicious anemia, nervousness, neuritis, fatigue, brain degeneration

Pangamic Acoid (B15 – not regarded as an essential B-vitamin)
Foods: In many vegetables and grains such as apricot kernels, brown rice, yeast, pumpkin and sunflower seeds.
Processes & Deficiency symptoms: While some claim benefits for a wide range of symptoms, diseases, and metabolic problems, there is limited information about deficiencies.

Laetrile (B17 – regarded as an essential B-vitamin)
Foods: Bitter almonds, further cores of stone fruits like peach, plum and apricot, large quantities of blue and green cassava and small quantities of cereals and pulses.
Processes: reducing the pain cause by arthritis, reduction/increase in blood pressure to its normal value
Deficiency symptoms: reduced resistance of a person's body against chronic diseases, such as cancer

Biotin (regarded as an essential B-vitamin)
Foods: Egg yolks, yeast, brown rice, soybeans, liver, kidney, sardines / mackerel (canned), royal jelly, walnuts, peanuts, mushrooms.
Processes: Fat, carbohydrate, & protein metabolism, fatty acid formation, helps utilize B vitamins;
Deficiency symptoms: Dry grayish skin, hair loss, scaly red rash around eyes-nose-mouth, depression, muscle pain, fatigue, poor appetite

Choline (not an official B-vitamin)
Foods: Organ meat, egg yolk, meat (muscle), fish, whole grain products, yeast, soy beans, lecithin, green vegetables.
Processes: Nerve transmission, fat & cholesterol metabolism, regulates liver & gall bladder
Deficiency symptoms: High blood pressure, bleeding stomach ulcers, liver & kidney problems

Vitamin C (Ascorbic Acid)
Foods: Broccoli, spinach, Brussels sprouts, cabbage, cauliflower, citrus fruits, strawberries and kiwi, rose hips, acerola cherries, black berries, red peppers, parsley, red cabbage, papaya, horseradish.
Processes: Wound healing, blood vessel strength, collagen maintenance, resistance to infection
Deficiency symptoms: Scurvy, bleeding gums, slow healing wounds, bruising, aching joints, nosebleeds, poor digestion

Vitamin E (Alfa-tocopherol)
Foods: Wheat Germ, (vegetable oils), soy, whole grain products, nuts, broccoli, spinach, butter, eggs, halibut, shrimp.

Processes: Cellular respiration, protects fat soluble vitamins & red blood cells, inhibits blood coagulation

Deficiency symptoms: Muscular wasting, abnormal fat deposits in muscles, gastrointestinal disease, heart disease

Citric acid
Foods: Primarily lemons and limes. The concentrations of citric acid in citrus fruits range from 0.005 mol/L for oranges and grapefruits to 0.30 mol/L in lemons and limes. You can find citric acid present in certain berries too, particularly raspberries and blackberries.

Processes: Citric acid bonds easily to minerals and metals, called chelation. It can help to take certain minerals with citric acid, since the body will more easily digest chelated minerals.

Deficiency symptoms: Although Dr. Moerman identified citric acid as one of the 8 essential nutrients, citric acid has no potential deficiencies or toxicities according to our current scientific evidence-base.

Iron (food must be very bad to have an iron deficiency occur)
Foods: Cornflakes, oat flakes, potatoes, liver, beef, soybeans, organ meats, chicken, eggs, parsley, mussels, oysters, nuts, sardines, spinach, sesame seeds, lentils, apple.

Processes: Carrier of oxygen to the tissues from the lungs in the form of hemoglobin, transport medium for electrons within the cells in the form of cytochromes, and an integral part of enzyme reactions in various tissues

Deficiency symptoms: Symptoms of iron deficiency are not unique to iron deficiency, but can include fatigue, dizziness, pallor, hair loss, irritability, weakness, brittle or grooved nails

Iodine
Foods: Fish, shellfish, seaweed (kelp), iodized salt, bread (iodized salt is incorporated into bread in the Netherlands - mandatory by Dutch Law for bakeries), fish (especially salmon, cod and haddock), cereals.

Processes: thyroid hormone production

Deficiency symptoms: Thyroid enlargement, mental imbalances such as depression and anxiety, mental retardation (in extreme cases, and particular in children of mothers who have had an iodine deficiency), fetal hypothyroidism (improper functioning of the thyroid in unborn children, leading to brain damage), autism, inability of the bodies organs to detoxify

Sulfur
Foods: Egg yolks, meat, fish, peppers, onions, beans, peas, leeks, garlic, cabbage, horseradish, Brussels sprouts.

Processes: Supporting aerobic metabolism, synthesis of protein and enzyme reactions, protection of joints, maintains the balance of oxygen in the body and keeps skin, hair and nails healthy, role in producing collagen

Deficiency symptoms: Pain and inflammation associated with various muscle and skeletal disorders, inflammation of the intestines associated with a wide range of symptoms, obesity, Crohn's disease, Alzheimer, heart disease, skin disorders, arthritis

Although Dr. Moerman did not call attention to additional vitamins, such as vitamin D and vitamin K, the food in his food plan amply covers these additional nutrients. The same can be said with regards to other minerals such as calcium, chromium, copper, magnesium, manganese, phosphorus, potassium, selenium and zinc.

However, for the sake of completeness, we include the additional vitamins and minerals below.

Vitamin D (Calciferal)
Foods: Egg yolk, herring, sardines (canned), shrimp, mackerel, fish oil, liver (tear), butter (fat) milk, cheese, brewer's yeast.

Processes: Bone formation, heart action, nervous system maintenance

Deficiency symptoms: Rickets, poor bone growth, nervous system irritability

Vitamin K
Foods: Cauliflower, cabbage, spinach, broccoli, lettuce, sprouts, green tea, molasses, cheese, eggs, butter, liver.

Processes: Formation of blood clotting agents

Deficiency symptoms: Tendency to hemorrhage

Calcium
Foods: Milk & milk products, dark green leafy vegetables, fortified foods

Processes: Strong bones, teeth, muscle tissue, regulates heart beat, muscle action & nerve functions, blood clotting

Deficiency symptoms: Soft, brittle bones, back & leg pain, heart palpitations, tetany

Chromium
Foods: Corn oil, clams, whole grain cereals, yeast
Processes: Glucose metabolism [energy], increases effectiveness of insulin
Deficiency symptoms: Atherosclerosis, glucose intolerance in diabetes

Copper
Foods: Oysters, nuts, organ meats, vegetables
Processes: Formation of red blood cells, bone growth & health, works with vitamin C to form elastin
Deficiency symptoms: General weakness, impaired respiration, skin sores

Magnesium
Foods: Nuts, seeds, green vegetables, whole grains
Processes: Acid/alkaline balance, metabolism of carbohydrates & minerals
Deficiency symptoms: Nervousness, tremors, easily aroused anger, disorientation, blood clots

Manganese
Foods: Nuts, whole grains, fruits, vegetables
Processes: Enzyme activation, fat & carbohydrate production, sex hormone production, skeletal development
Deficiency symptoms: Dizziness, poor muscle coordination, tinnitus (ear noises)

Phosphorus
Foods: Fish, meat, poultry, eggs, whole grains
Processes: Bone development, important in fat, protein, & carbohydrate utilization
Deficiency symptoms: Poor bones & teeth, arthritis, rickets, appetite loss, irregular breathing

Potassium
Foods: Lean meats, vegetables, fruits
Processes: Fluid balance, control activity of heart muscle, nervous system, kidneys
Deficiency symptoms: Poor reflexes, irregular heartbeat, dry skin, general weakness

Selenium
Foods: Seafood, organ meats, lean meats, whole grains, Brazil nuts, eggs

Processes: Protects body tissues against oxidation damage from radiation, pollution & normal metabolic processing
Deficiency symptoms: Heart muscle abnormalities

Zinc
Foods: Lean meats, liver, eggs, seafood, whole grains
Processes: Involved in digestion & metabolism, important in development of reproductive systems, aids in healing
Deficiency symptoms: Retarded growth, prolonged wound healing, loss of appetite

When (small) clinical symptoms persist and endure

We will develop one or more clinical symptoms time and again during the course of our lives. I most certainly developed a lot of them in the years preceding my cancer. When we deal with them promptly there really aren't any grounds for concern. But when we ignore them or push them aside with patchwork medications and remedies, they may return and start to haunt us with increasing regularity and growing intensity. As the body's self-healing abilities become over-taxed, so the symptoms will return more frequently and more severely, until a point is reached when we are suffering from a few of these symptoms simultaneously and we find ourselves on the brink of a chronic illness such as cancer.

When these symptoms start to persist, then we are witnessing a gradual breakdown of our immune system. When we choose to ignore these early warning signals, allowing them to continue for months and years on end (it's amazing how much our bodies can actually endure) then we can reach a point where our body is forced to declare a state of emergency and switch to a last-resort survival mode.

In simple terms, we will have reached a complex state of being where different body organs are suffering from (partial) damage, overloading, constrained inflows and outflows. When this happens, our whole body system has effectively been derailed. Nutritional material is not reaching the places where it is needed, and starts to accumulate in all sorts of nooks and crannies. Acid crystals in the joints. Sugars, starches and salts start to accumulate on roadsides all over the place, particularly on congested roads around the cities, which in our bodies are represented by major vital organs, e.g. brain, lungs, liver, kidneys, stomach, bladder, and the lymphatic system organs such as the spleen, thymus and lymph nodes.

There comes a do-or-die point where our body either collapses under this strain, or makes one final attempt to buy some extra time. Cancer buys us this extra time, setting up temporary storage dumps where they are needed. Local storage points where waste is gathered and contained. These storage locations are the cancer tumors.

A closing thought

We are complex beings with a network of processing centers and distribution channels, with input and output points connecting us to the physical and non-physical world in which we exist. And as is the case in complex logistics networks, seemingly innocent difficult-to-measure breakdowns that can occur unnoticed in less traveled areas, only become apparent when they unexpectedly lead to larger setbacks in critical processes and distribution channels. Striving for a balanced co-operation between all involved parts should be our goal, and being alert to early warning signals is an essential component.

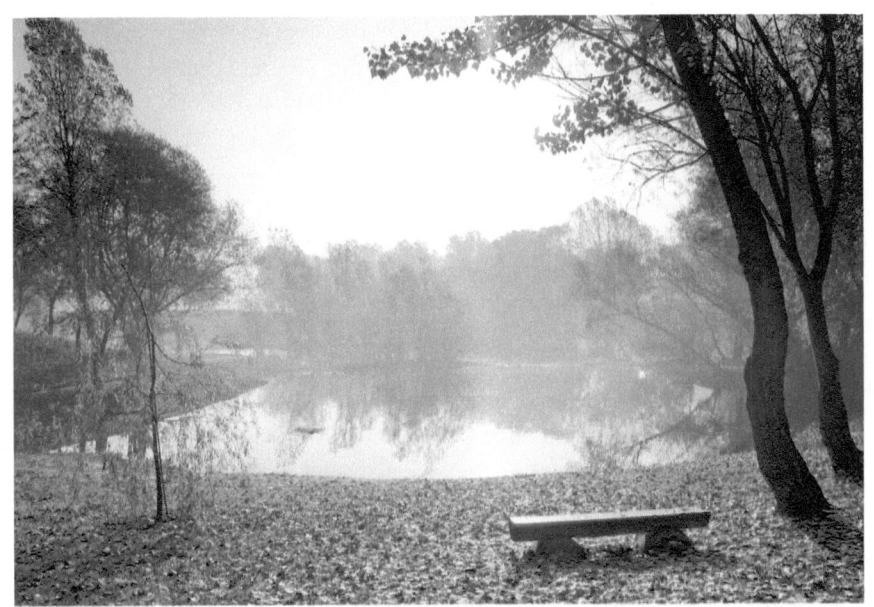

2 GOOD FOOD

One fact that there is across-the-board agreement on is: cancer thrives when there are high levels of sugar in the blood. This leads to the notion that sugar "feeds" cancer tumors. I choose my words carefully, because the actual "feeding" relationship between blood sugar and cancer tumors has still to be determined.

Nevertheless, the food plan that can stabilize the blood sugar levels is characterized by:

- low intake of processed foods that are high in refined flours and sugars;
- low intake of foods that are high in white starches (sugar, white flour, potatoes);
- high intake of foods that are close to their original forms found in nature (whole fruits, whole grains, whole vegetables);

- look for colorful (anti-inflammatory) produce such as blueberries, cruciferous vegetables (broccoli, cauliflower) and tomatoes;
- consume naturally healthy fats found in nuts, seeds, (coco)nut butters, extra-virgin olive oil, canola oil, and avocados;
- limit alcohol consumption to one to two glasses per day; red wine is the best choice, since it has the most anti-inflammatory chemicals.

These food plan characteristics are a useful first step towards developing, what I have chosen to call, a liver-friendly food plan.

When the liver is healthy, i.e. clean and functioning well within its design limits, it is difficult for cancer to get out of control. I would like to say impossible for cancer to get out of control, but nature is always able to produces exceptions to the rule.

When cancer has grown out of control, the liver is usually at the limits of its ability to perform the functions it was designed for. The liver may be damaged. It will almost certainly be overloaded. And it will most certainly be far from clean. Unable to perform its basic functions will results in other organs and bodily processes starting to malfunction. Natural flows become interrupted. The ability to absorb nutrients and the ability to dispose of wastes is hampered. The body systems start to clog up. One popular abstract description is that our immune system starts to "break down" or "derail" so that we are no longer able to contain the cancer in our bodies. In short, our liver is overworked and overloaded.

The three key lifestyle changes, including good food, are designed to help us unclog the system and get things flowing again. So good food is not only about nutrition. It is also about reducing the load on our liver. Together with sleep and exercise it is also about stimulating the liver to start cleaning up the mess and get things flowing again. There is plenty to clean up, especially when you consider that the cancer-out-of-control state has been building up over a period of many years. This makes it all the more amazing when we realize that the house cleaning operation can be performed inside 4-6 weeks.

The lack of energy and lack of appetite sometimes associated with cancer patients leads to one categorical imperative for a food plan: restore a clean liver and keep it clean. This implies that when it is difficult to consume fruits and vegetables in their natural state, they should be blended into a mushy pulp or juice that can be served with a spoon. If the fibers and pulp are still difficult to consume, then they should be extracted with a juicing machine so that only the liquid is left. Don't compound the challenge of overcoming a lack of appetite by serving the cancer patient water alone, or teas and broths with little to no nutritional content. They fill the stomach, thus making it more difficult for the cancer patient to consume the life saving nutrition he/she needs. In the worst case scenarios, the cancer patient is fed vegetable juices, freshly obtained from a juicing machine, one spoonful at a time. In the worst case scenario, we would start with juices of carrots and broccoli, and as the cancer patient improves, expand with more varieties of vegetables and fruits.

I was fortunate enough to still have a good appetite in my early days with cancer, so food consumption was not an issue. But had I suffered from a loss of appetite, then a few spoonfuls of vegetable juice would not have contained the essential nutrition required to maintain a healthy body. In that case I would have been dealing with a sick body that required a gentle kick-start of the liver functions by first entering a cleansing (detoxification) phase. My body would have been so clogged up, especially the digestive track, that many of the essential nutrients would not be absorbed anyway, and just pile up as even more waste to be disposed of – additional load for the liver functions. This is something that I will now keep in mind when someone recommends force feeding a cancer patient. I now realize that force-feeding just for the sake of feeding is not a good idea, because the body and the liver need to go through an initial detoxification process first.

The fresh juices provide the essential starting fuel to get the fire of life going again – to gently stimulate the liver into action. Some researchers attribute this to phytochemicals (chemicals that plants produce to protect themselves, that possibly/probably also help us to protect our bodies against disease) and talk about foods that fight cancer. Others emphasize the benefits of vitamin C. And others talk about the effects of enzymes that are released in raw food when freshly juiced or blended or chewed in the mouth. And others place emphasis on absence of the poisoned foods that the cancer patient normally consumed, the absence of the excess sugar and salt and other chemical additives found in factory processed foods – overheated in the canning process, the dead foods, the foods of death, the foods that serve to clog up the system and overload the liver. The truth is probably all of the above and much more that continues to elude us, because it lies beyond the current capabilities of our scientific evidence-based research.

Should I ever find myself in a desperate situation with cancer again, bed-ridden, no energy and no appetite, then my path back is crystal clear: raw fruits and vegetables, freshly blended, freshly juiced, consumed gently spoonful by spoonful, sipped gently, chewed gently... my first gentle steps along the path back to recovery can be this simple.

Armed with this basic understanding, I would then move into the Moerman type food plan as a whole. And allow my level of appetite to dictate how I evolved my own food plan during the course of the first 4-6 weeks. In case of doubt, *a little less* is better than *a little more*. I will be gentle on myself.

The food plan for cancer patients

I made my food plan really simple, by identifying what I should and what I should not buy in the shops:

YES to whole foods: fruits including seeds and skins, whole grains, whole vegetables
YES to raw foods
YES to foods that have only been cold pressed (oils), naturally dried (fruits) or mechanically ground (whole grains)
YES to farm products such as buttermilk and eggs
YES to sources for proteins such as seeds, beans and grains, fruits such as goji berries, quinoa, amaranth, brown rice, mungo beans and farm products such as egg yolks and buttermilk
NO to water (water just fills the stomach and takes away appetite needed for other foods that provide essential nutrition): fluid to be obtained from fruits and vegetables and farm products such as buttermilk
NO to meat, NO to fish (too much effort required from body and liver to process the proteins)
NO to foods that have gone through a chemical process or heating process as is the case in food factories
NO to foods that have had part of the original food removed, often the seeds or skins, such as white rice, white flour, split peas, tomato puree
NO to foods that have a high sugar or starch content, e.g. dates and potatoes
NO to foods that have a high salt content, e.g. salted butter and cheese
NO to foods containing processed fats such as cheese and margarine

I used the check list above to design and build my own liver-friendly food plan. In the following section I share my thoughts on the design of a liver-friendly food plan. At the end of the chapter I delve into a more detailed check list for the food plan I built for myself.

Designing my liver-friendly food plan

What constitutes a liver-friendly food plan? An even simpler question I started with was "what is liver-friendly food?"

As I have previously mentioned in this chapter, my own learning process started with the work of Dr. Moerman. He had identified 8 essential nutrients that were essential to restoring the balance in a healthy body and immune system, and should therefore be present in our daily food: vitamin A, vitamin C, vitamin E, citric acid, yeast (we now refer to this as the whole complex of vitamin B), iron, iodine and sulfur.

My understanding is that these nutrients were regarded by Dr. Moerman as essential for maintaining a healthy body, a body free of the small clinical symptoms, a body in which the cancer process is under control, a body that resist infections such as colds and flu's, a body that can recover quickly from accidental damage or short-term abuse (lack of sleep, intense training, long business trip.) He had identified the small clinical symptoms that indicated a deficiency in one or more of these essential nutrients, which led to the development of the Moerman food plan.

It may well be that these 8 nutrients, and the underlying synergy that exists between them, are indeed the key to a healthy body. Part of this key may may also be that the scala of whole foods containing these essential nutrients also contain other essential (micro)nutrients that nature has designed into these foods – an additional dimension to the food synergy network. Additional factors can be the manner in which we combine different foods and prepare our food.

I developed a rough list for myself, in which I listed the 8 essential nutrients (and a few more) identified by Dr. Moerman. For each nutrient I listed the foods that contained this nutrient, which body processes utilized this nutrient, and last but not least which small clinical symptoms might be associated with a deficiency. This is the list I included in the previous chapter.

My sole purpose was to see if my daily food plan was well balanced and perhaps identify a handful of simple foods that I would consume on a daily basis.

The handful of simple foods that I use daily in my food plan have stabilized over time. On any particular day I may add more fruits and vegetables and nuts and seeds for variety, but the foods below are included each and every day:

- lemons
- virgin olive oil
- egg yolks
- home baked bread (whole grain spelt, pumpkin seeds, iodized salt, yeast)
- home baked goji bread (whole grain spelt, goji berries, figs, Brazil nuts, yeast)
- salads and juices containing red onions, leafy dark green vegetables (lettuce, spinach, spring onions, broccoli), tomatoes, carrots
- fatty fish (salmon, herring, mackerel)
- butter-milk
- goji berries

There is nothing special about these foods over other alternative foods. Or maybe there is. Either way, they just happen to be the foods that I habitually buy and consume daily. And they just happen to amply cover all the essential and non-essential nutrients I write about in this chapter.

The whole food or just the juice?

And as we have learned from the introduction to this chapter, the whole food can be consumed if the cancer patient's appetite allows it. But in cases of poor appetite, then the raw fruits and vegetables should be juiced for the patient, thereby removing the pulp which usually means removing the fibers, seeds and skins. Note that when the cancer patient can stomach it (interesting expression), then the fibers can be included for their "roughage" quality, and seeds and skins as well for their added nutritional value.

However, I also came to realize that when the seeds and skins are exposed to the blades of a kitchen blender or juicing machine, the resulting process of cutting and grinding also releases some of the nutrients in the seeds and skins into the juice.

How do these guidelines translate to specific foods?

The yolks of eggs are full of nutrients, and easy to digest and absorb. They lend themselves to mixing into sauces, or dressings such as mayonnaise. This way they can be eaten raw. The white of the egg should be cooked, e.g in soft boiled eggs, but is a little more difficult to consume. Where possible, stick to the raw egg-yolk only.

The only dairy products I recommend are buttermilk that is still made on the farm.

Plenty of fresh fruit and vegetables and freshly pressed juices. Mixing with buttermilk into smoothies for added variety. I consume the juice of 5-6 lemons each day, as juices, in smoothies, in the salad dressing, in mayonnaise. My vegetables I eat raw as well both in the form of salads as well as run through the kitchen blender to produce a sort of guacamole. And when so inclined, I will run them through the juicing machine thereby removing the pulp and leaving the juice, and try out new recipes by mixing them into my smoothies.

I try to work cold pressed oils into most of my meals. Olive oil goes into my salads and soups. Flex (linseed) oil goes into my smoothies.

Add variety to the raw vegetables by including those seeds and beans that can be sprouted (germinated) at home.

When your appetite is good, you can start to include "heated" food. For me they are home baked bread, pizza's, soup broths with unpolished (brown) rice or quinoa, and soups with blended vegetables. For bread and pizza bottoms I have found that of all the whole grains, the spelt appears to digest most easily. I only include these foods to add to the variety. At least 80-90% of what I eat and drink is raw food. During my first 6 weeks 100% was raw.

There's a reason Popeye's girl friend was named Olive Oyl

Spinach and olive oil belong together. The fat in the oil releases the nutrients in the spinach and makes them more bio-available (easier to digest and absorb the nutrients), and the two create a terrific taste when used together. The idea that "the fat in the oil releases nutrients" appeals to my imagination and justifies the thought that cold-pressed olive oils combined with food have, throughout the ages, been regarded as healthy in the French, Spanish, Italian and Greek kitchens and the kitchens of other countries around the world where olive trees flourished..

The lemon & extra virgin olive oil drink

I quickly developed an intuitive habit of mixing lemon juice and olive oil into my meals. It started off as a dressing for the salads, but I habitually add it to soups and pizza's as well.

I also developed the habit of starting the day off with the juice of one lemon in a glass of warm water. After more reading and research I modified this habit by using the whole lemon (no waxed skin and thoroughly cleaned.) What I now do is cut one lemon into small pieces, add about a table spoon of extra virgin olive oil, add some warm water and run this through the kitchen blender. I then pour it through a strainer thereby removing the pulp.

The lemon (including the lemon rind and seeds) and extra virgin olive oil, when taken together, and diluted to taste with some warm water, can act as a potent liver and gallbladder flush. This can set off a whole scala of desirable and related causes and effects. These include detoxifying the liver., lowering biliruben levels, removing heavy metals, increasing the production of bile from the liver, stimulating lymphatic flow, and restoring the pH of your saliva, which in turn helps you to absorb the nutrients from the food you eat.

The liver is truly the master organ of the immune system, producing chemicals to combat viruses (including the HIV virus) and bacteria, supporting phagocytic [immune function], and producing antihistamines to neutralize substances that promote the growth of cancer. When the liver is not functioning properly - and is over-blocked by toxins - the body's immune system is severely weakened leading to chronic illness. The lemon & extra virgin olive oil drink can both prevent chronic illness as well as work to reverse it.

Take care of your liver

At the risk of over-simplification, if you want to prevent cancer, protect your liver. When you have cancer, you know that your liver is screwed up. But your liver possesses two unique and useful qualities. It has a huge overcapacity for performing the functions it was designed for. And it has the ability to regenerate itself. When nature bestows these "super" qualities to one of our body organs, we should treat this organ with the respect it deserves.

Books have been written about the human liver. There is a saying that you look as old or as young as your liver is clean. The liver is the great orchestrator of hundreds, if not thousands, of body functions that include keeping our blood clean, removing pollutants before they have a chance to congregate throughout our body, removing dead or damaged blood cells from circulation, storage of nutrients and release of these nutrients as and when they are needed, storing extra blood for emergencies, helping to keep blood sugar levels stable, helping to break down fats, etc. The heart is the endurance runner, but the liver is the work horse that keeps our bodies clean even when subjected to high loads under extreme conditions. But there is a limit to what the liver can do, and as this limit is approached we witness a gradual accumulation of the early warning signals (the small clinical symptoms), and when this limit is reached, we witness the appearance of chronic diseases such as cancer.

This is why the three key lifestyle changes can reap immediate benefits within weeks, if not days. The initial detox/cleanup bring the demands on the liver down to a level within its design capacity, and at the same time the reduced load on the liver means that the liver has the opportunity to start regenerating. Once this turning point is reached, improvements start to kick in throughout the body, as the liver is able to role up its sleeves and clean house, and the increased sense of well being and returning vitality make themselves evident.

These are just some of the many questions that one can raise on this subject:

- Which food can best be consumed when?
- Should one eat and drink at the same time?
- Is it wise to mix various food groups in one meal?
- Should one avoid eating in-between meals?

- Is a warm meal better than a cold one?

Below is a simple, compact guideline that I drew up for myself. Whenever I use the expression "try to" it's because I personally tend to do it "most of the time." In theory, in a perfect world, I would love to be able to do it "all of the time", but my life just does not work that way.

- All food processing (cooking) should be kept to a minimum. Food should be consumed as fresh as possible.
- Fruits and vegetables (whenever possible) should be unsprayed and grown without chemical fertilizers.
- The meal should be consumed in a relaxed manner. When feeling agitated or rushed, you are better off consuming as little as possible.
- Chew your food well before consuming and drink slowly. Why? The saliva you produce is essential to a healthy digestion process.
- Try to start each morning off with the freshly squeezed juice of a lemon in a glass of warm water, or go for the more potent liver and gallbladder flush that entails using the whole lemon and extra virgin olive oil. Your liver will thank you for it.
- Stick to fruit and vegetable juices (with moderate use of buttermilk, flax-seed oil) for the remainder of the morning until noon.
- Restrict your drinking during meals to a small glass of e.g. red wine, buttermilk or green tea.
- Keep your meals as simple as possible (single course) and try not to mix too many different food groups in the same meal, e.g. no fruit desert after a bread or rice meal.
- Try to eat/drink at regular intervals of 2 hours.
- Try to finish eating by 7pm. Consume only water or green tea after that. Try to observe a 12 hour overnight period of fasting.
- Try to get to bed by 9pm. A warm water bottle resting against your liver is a welcome aid during periods of body detoxification/cleansing.
- Try to get to sleep by 10pm. Your sleep between 10pm - 2pm is critical for body healing and rebuilding processes.

I am fully aware from personal experience how challenging this sleeping schedule can be, as it interferes with a normal social family and working life. But the choice was mine and mine alone. I could have chosen for the more socially acceptable route of the social get-together, meals and snacks and

TV watching into the later hours of the evening, and watch my planned daily routine disintegrate in a puff of smoke. Or I could choose for life, and do what needed to be done, for myself and for my family.

Cod-liver oil

Take a look at the old fisherman and his wife. See what a beneficial effect fish oils have had on their lives. Some will sing the praises of the daily fish oil or cod liver oil supplements. And today's oils taste much better than that ghastly stuff our mother's used to spoon-feed us with back in the 1950s. Maybe the fish oil supplementation did contribute to the health and long life of the old fisherman and his wife. But somebody else might point out that their life was not an easy life – simple yes, but easy no. They both had to get up early in the morning and start laboring over fish net repairs, cleaning the boat, getting the tackle ready, preparing meals, taking the boat out, working the boat, unloading the boat, cleaning the fish, etc. It was not an easy life, but it was a physically active life from early morning to early bed times. And as far as the cod liver oil is concerned, this old fisherman recalls how they fermented their cod liver oil in casks, a natural process that took about half a year, but then you had quality stuff. He turns up his nose at the stuff we call cod liver oil today. A faster and cheaper factory heating process has replaced the natural time-consuming fermentation, and the resulting oil has no taste and little of it's original medicinal properties remain. But what do an old fisherman and his wife know about modern food production processes and the results of scientific evidence-based research?

No meat – no fish

No meat and no fish for the cancer patient! Oh? Are meat and fish not healthy? They are both sources of protein, and the body can certainly use some protein. The meat protein is more difficult to digest and absorb than the fish protein, which in turn is more difficult to digest and absorb than protein obtained from dairy products such as buttermilk, egg yokes, grains, vegetables and fruits. Difficult translates into more effort (energy) and e.g. loading of the liver. And meat and fish come with much "accompanying body" that also translates into more processing and waste disposal loading.

Goji berries – super-food?

The fresh goji berry is packed-full with all the essential amino acids (protein), huge doses of vitamin C, and a long list of vitamins and minerals that are good for us. And sooner or later you will come across the story of the Chinese gentlemen who lived to the ripe old age of 200 years (this figure varies according to the source of the story). Observers noted that he ate a handful of goji berries each day, and naturally labeled the goji berry a superfood, and further research seems to support this. But other observers noted that this Chinese gentleman, needing to get away from the wife and screaming kids, both of which he had many during the course of his life. He would leave the house early each morning and pursue his 5 mile walk up the mountain trail. Taking his time, he enjoyed the walk for the pleasant pursuit it was, until he reached the goji orchard, where he would pick a handful of fresh berries. He would then sit down, relax, and eat his goji berries one by one, playing around with each berry in his mouth, taking the time to observe its taste and texture, swallowing gently and waiting a moment before proceeding to the next berry. By the time he finished consuming the last berry, it was time to rejoin the mountain trail and commence the return walk to his house... just in time for lunch with the family.

Good sources of protein (amino acids)

Seriously, goji berries are attributed with some 15-20% protein content, with all the essential amino acids, but so are the super foods of South America and India. The quinoa and amaranth seeds were to the Aztecs and Incas, what rice is to the Chinese, and what the mung bean is to people from India. Quinoa, amaranth and the mung bean are attributed with some 20% protein (once again, the actual figure varies according to the source).

Sprout your own food

My personal favorites are quinoa and mung beans, because I can sprout these seeds and beans in my kitchen. Much in the same way that I prefer broccoli sprouts to the full grown broccoli. In fact sprouts of any kind hold a favorite place on my food plate, because the sprouts are young, packed with nutrients, much easier to digest and absorb than their older brothers, and bursting with enzymes. Young and fresh translate into enzyme-rich in my vocabulary. And enzyme-rich translates into easy to digest and absorb. Just what the cancer patient needs – nutrition that is easy to digest and absorb.

Sprouting can be done within the confines of your own kitchen. It requires little space. You are effectively growing your own food. You don't have to invest in a garden, gardening tools or manure. You don't have to strain your back weeding. And beyond buying your seeds and beans in a grocery store, it doesn't cost you a cent extra. Welcome news in these challenging economic times.

The color code

As far as the saying "variety is the spice of life" goes, I stopped counting calories and checking all the different vitamins, minerals, carbohydrates, phytochemicals that I should be consuming each day in a so-called healthy food plan. I know which foods to eat. I know which foods to avoid. I am aware of the consequences of eating something from my forbidden list.

To make life easy for myself I quickly (intuitively at the beginning) adopted a color-code when shopping for my groceries. Apples: the insides represent white, but the skins represent red and green. The intenser the skin colors, the better in my book. Oranges represent orange. So do carrots. Lemons represent yellow. Spring onions represent white and green. Red onions actually represent purple, as do beets. Various lettuces represent green and purple. Paprikas come in red, yellow and green. The red strawberries, the purple blackberries, the different shades and tints of the raspberries and other berries. The fresh goji berry is actually a bright orange. The different shades of green in fresh herbs.

Simply put, different colors represent different nutrients or groups of nutrients. By covering all the colors of the rainbow, both when shopping as well as preparing meals and drinks (smoothies), I kind of ensure that I am getting the full range of nutrients into the food plan. For example, when preparing a salad or a smoothie, I am thinking white, yellow, green, red, orange and purple. This may not qualify as a scientific evidence-based approach, but it is a lot easier than thinking in terms of all the different nutrients I should be squeezing into my food plan.

I was doing this long before I studied for and qualified as a nutritionist. This was also before I learned about the latest research into curcumin, olive oil and black pepper, apricot pits, tomatoes heated in olive oil, quark mixed with flex oil, shi-take mushrooms, green tea, quinoa, goji berries and all the other natural food sources of special nutrients that supposedly fight cancer. At the very least research is trying to build on a correlative relationship between the presence of these food (combinations) in the meals we consume and the prevention and control of the cancer process.

One of the reasons that I am reluctant to buy into the foods that fight cancer approach is the simple fact that (most of, if not all of) these exotic foods were for many centuries only available to local populations, with their respective cultures and climates. I choose to think that each geographic location was (still is) capable of supplying a full range of foods to cover the nutritional requirements for healthy living. Having ready access to other foods imported from neighboring regions and abroad just gives us more choice and variety throughout the seasons.

So yes, we may identify the so-called super-foods and credit them with distinguishing nutritional features, but they are not essential for our daily food plan. My daily shopping is simple yet varied, and I manage a tight budget. In fact the cost of food for my family has dropped considerably since all the meat and fish and factory processed foods have disappeared from the shopping list. Naturally I tried out the super-foods for a while, and I still do now and again. They are "nice for a change" but not essential.

Should we go biological?

In the Netherlands we use the term "biological food" which is synonymous with organic food. From our personal health point of view the emphasis is simply on quality food, organic or otherwise. Each of us has to judge the reliability of the local organic label. And there are fruits and vegetables which both look good as well as taste good, and are produced locally, although they have not been stamped organic. Another factor that may affect our buying decisions is price. Additional considerations include animal and environmental friendliness.

Building my liver-friendly food plan

This liver-friendly food plan is my liver-friendly food plan, and even I only consider it as a general guideline or check-list. It is a repetition of what I have already written, presented in a format similar to the one used by Dr. Moerman. The rational behind what to eat or drink and what not to eat or drink can be found throughout the previous pages of this chapter.

The following list continues to serve me well as a check list. There is no particular order to the items on this check list. For a more simple check list I refer you, the reader, back to the YES / NO list at the beginning of this chapter.

No meat, fish or poultry. As an alternative source of protein use goji berries, quinoa, amaranth, brown rice, mung beans. Because of a good appetite, I allow myself fatty fish in moderation such as salmon, mackerel and herring.

Eggs may be eaten daily. Soft boiled. Use by preference uncooked egg-yolk as in salad dressings, mayonnaise.

No milk. Buttermilk daily.

A little young, low-salt, low-fat cheese.

A little unsalted butter..

No cream. No sour-cream.

Fruit and fruit juices daily. Preferably freshly blended, juiced or pressed.

Recommended for juice: lemon, grapefruit, apple, and oranges, and all sorts of berries (nutrient rich seeds and skins).

Preferably with juicing machine or blender/strainer, so that nutrients in seeds and skins are also extracted into the juice.

Recommended fresh fruit: pineapple, grapefruit, kiwi, avocado, mango and papaya.

In moderation apricots, raisins, dried or fresh figs, dried or fresh goji berries. No dates.

Fresh, raw vegetables daily. Juiced, blended or cut in salads. All vegetables can be juiced, especially when appetite is poor. I have a juice maker, but I am reluctant to use it because cleaning out the residue pulp is time consuming. The juice maker works best for vegetables such as carrots and broccoli, but I use a kitchen blender followed by a strainer for fruits, such as my lemon/olive oil drink in the morning.

Recommended raw vegetables: broccoli, cabbages, soya beans, pulse, tomatoes, carrots, beetroot, onions and garlic and all the dark green leafy varieties such as spinach, lettuces, spring onions, leek.

Vegetable soups in moderation.

Recommended soup vegetables: just about any vegetable, such as peas, carrots, onions, leek, broccoli, tomatoes, garlic, lentils. Goes well with my spelt bread. And when I do not feel like eating my egg yolks raw, I mix them into my bowl of soup.

No potatoes.

In moderation bread. I have two basic recipes (1) whole grain, preferably spelt, with pumpkin seeds and Brazil nuts, and yeast and a pinch of iodized salt, and (2) whole grain, preferably spelt, with goji berries, Brazil nuts, figs and yeast and optionally one or two teaspoons of honey.

In moderation whole grain rice. Excellent alternatives are quinoa and amaranth, which contain all the essential amino acids (proteins).

Flour products in moderation. Only whole grain, preferably spelt.

Spaghetti and other pastas in moderation. Only whole grain, preferably spelt.

Germinated seeds and grains are not a must, but they are excellent sources of "young" and "vital" nutrition.

Only cold pressed oils such as linseed oil and extra virgin olive oil. These oils, when added to salads and soups (low temperature heat) and juices, make it easier for the body to extract and absorb the nutrition in the food. No peanut oil and no aragis oil.

Nuts in moderation. Recommended are hazelnuts, almonds, walnuts, Brazil nuts. No peanuts. In moderation hazelnut oil and almond oil, which are not quite cold-pressed, as a little warming up is required to extract the oil.

Sunflower seeds, pumpkin seeds, linseed and sesame-seeds.

Herbs are strongly recommended, especially when they are fresh and of the dark green leafy varieties such as basil and chives. Sliced tomatoes, basil, mozzarella cheese and virgin green olive oil is a favorite salad prepared in minutes.

Any herbs are allowed, even recommended. Spices in general not allowed.

Spices. With the exception of black pepper, spices are generally not recommended.

For sweetening purposes use one or two teaspoons per day of good quality honey. No refined sugar and no sugar replacements.

No salt, except in bread and cheese.

No foods that have been factory processed in any way, including heated, refined, canned, preserved.

Not permitted.

Coffee and tea in moderation. Preferably a green tea.

No cocoa.

Try to avoid drinking water alone. Preferred sources are fruits, vegetables and butter-milk, and water used in soups and teas.

Biological, dynamic/organic products are preferred. I still manage to find very good fruits and vegetables that do not carry a biological label.

No alcohol, with the exception of one or two glasses of red wine with a meal.

At least 80% of what I eat and drink is raw. The breads are baked, omelets are prepared in olive oil with a little butter (short low-temperature heating), the soups are gently boiled for 3-5 minutes and then blended. I don't like cooking my vegetables for longer periods of time, and I don't like the higher temperatures associated with pressure cookers and steaming. No microwave. No re-heating cooked food.

Special note on "cold" foods

I have always consumed raw foods, fruit juices, vegetable juices and buttermilk at room temperature. On hindsight this was intuitive at best, most probably coincidental, and certainly not by design.

Because I drink freshly squeezed juices of fruits and vegetables, the raw juices are consumed at room temperature.

The buttermilk that I mix into my breakfast or smoothies is at room temperature by the time I consume it.

All the raw vegetables that go into salads, even those stored in the fridge, are at room temperature by the time they have been prepared, brought to the table and are ready for consumption.

Are foods and drinks that have been stored in the fridge and consumed directly at "cold" temperatures detrimental to one's health, i.e. taxing on the liver and the digestive process? My intuition appears to have said yes, but my honest answer: I have no idea. On a hot summer day I still enjoy an ice-cold drink, be it from the fridge or from a mountain stream, and this time by design.

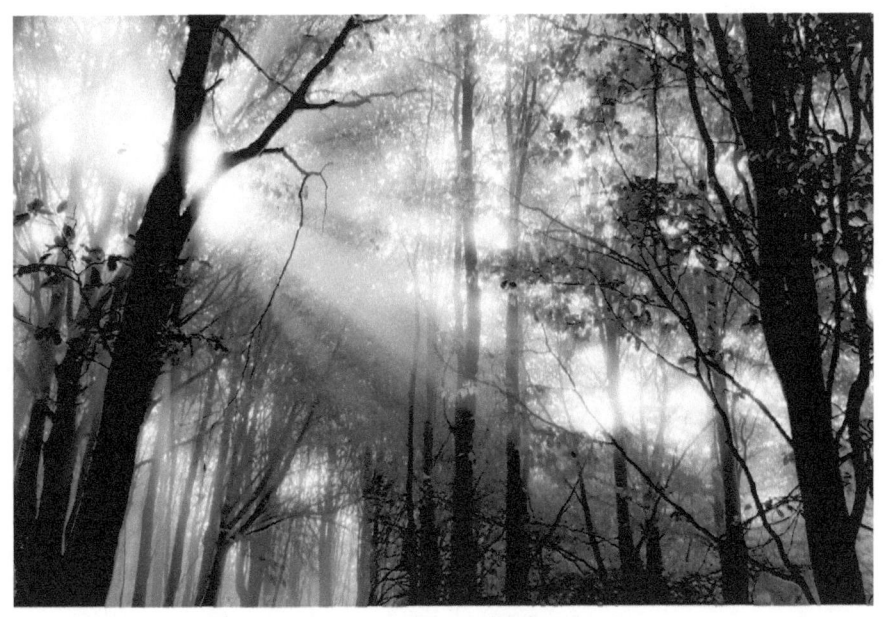

3 GENTLE EXERCISE

My early morning walk

My first 10 walks behind me. 10 different walks.
My first 100 walks behind me. 100 different walks.
My first 1000 walks behind me. 1000 different walks.
Slow walks and brisk walks.
Some walks breaking into gentle runs.
Some walks shorter, some walks longer.
Barefoot walks and trail shoe walks.
Walks in the rain, walks in the snow.
Walks in the early morning sun, walks in the mist.
Walks in the forest, walks in the mountains.
Walks in the countryside and walks on the beach.
Chi walks and power walks.
Walks filled with flowing thoughts.
Walks filled with emotional outbursts.

Walks filled with new insights and inspiration.
Walks filled with stories to be told.
Walks filled with my surroundings.
Walks filled with sounds.
Walks filled with sights.
Walks filled with smells.
Walks filled with silence.
Walks filled with hand energy flowing.
Walks filled with rhythmic breathing.
Nose breathing in, nose breathing out.
Nose breathing in, mouth breathing out.
Stomach muscles expanding, stomach muscles contracting.
Walks filled with passing glimpses of foxes.
Walks filled with bird calls.
The deer – gracefully, silently gliding over the path before me.
The fox – frozen one moment, gone the next.
Magical moments of awareness – part of me forever.

Some of the questions I asked myself

45 minutes each day in the countryside/forest... can I fit that into my busy life? For me it has become a top priority, and during my first 3 months as a cancer patient I only missed one day.

Do I cycle to and from work alongside roads packed with car traffic? How healthy is that compared to a brisk walk in the forest? When I bicycle into town in the afternoons to do some shopping at the health store, I now take the cycle paths through the forest.

Do I jog a few times per week in the vicinity of (car) exhaust fumes? How relaxing is that compared to a brisk walk in the countryside? Well, I am inclined to break into a gentle run when the mood grabs me, but I avoid walking alongside traffic as much as possible.

Once again the emphasis is on quality as opposed to quantity.

I strive to walk each day:

- briskly for 45 minutes with a heart rate of 100-120 beats per minute;
- in the early morning sun (rainy days are OK as well);

- in the local forest which is an oxygen rich environment;
- soaking up the here and now of the forest life (sight, sound, smells);
- letting my thoughts bubble to the surface as and when they arise;
- reflecting on thoughts, emotions... anything goes;
- playing around with breathing exercises.

My morning walk is a time of exercise, meditation, self reflection, focus, concentration and relaxation. It is a vital part of my day. And yes, there are times that I get to bed a little late, get up next morning a little late, and my morning walk gets shifted to the afternoon or the evening. And it is not long before I see the structure of may daily routines start to crumble, until I go off on my early morning walk again the next day, and then the next, and I see the structure return.

Along the way I discovered my morning walk to be my personal key that opens the door to the structure of my daily routine. This is not a walk with friends, or an hour's cycling, or a round of golf. This is my walk, alone, in a natural environment filled only with the sounds and sights and smells of nature. Filled with the magical moments of awareness – physically, mentally, emotionally. And on occasion spiritually.

Beyond gentle exercise

There comes a point in time when we have recovered from cancer sufficiently to warrant more intensive exercise and training, particularly if we participate in competitive sports or simply enjoy running, cycling, squash, golf, etc.

My daily routine always ensured that my meals or drinks took place within an hour of exercising, e.g. breakfast around 7.30am after a morning walk from say 6-7am, or a protein rich goji-berry smoothie within an hour of completing a 2 hour cycling session. When I started exercising more intensely, such as training for an endurance cycling event in the first half of 2011, I tended to recover better and more quickly from the daily training routine whenever I ate my meals (or drank my energy smoothies) within 1 hour of completing the training session. It felt as if my body was in a much better state to process the meals and absorb the nutrition. Bottom line: a reduced load on the liver and maximum absorption of nutrition.

I may not be able to provide the scientific evidence-base to back up this anecdote, yet intuitively it all makes perfect sense to me.

Closing thoughts on my early morning walk

My early morning walk plays such an important, essential role in my daily life. It is a way for me to stimulate my liver into action before breakfast and the challenges of the new day. It is a way to gently massage my lymphatic organs with the up and down motion of my walk. It is a way to breathe new life into my body. It is a way to remind myself that new life can only be breathed in when wasted or spent life is breathed out. It is a time of day when thoughts and emotions are given the opportunity to bubble to the surface. This has nothing to do with good or bad emotions, or whether I should or should not be thinking this way or that. Every thought has the right to exist. It exists for a reason. Every emotion has the right to exist. It exists for a reason. Some thoughts and emotions need to be dealt with. They ask for awareness and attention. Others are ready to be released. Time to let them go and move on.

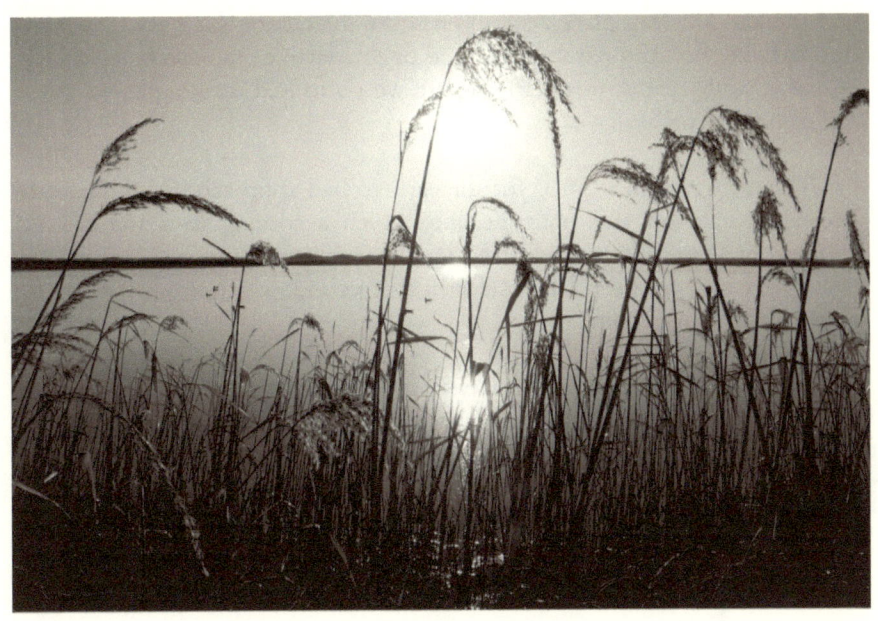

4 SLEEPING WELL

Colon cleansing and liver cleansing

This may seem a strange way to start a chapter on sleeping, but there is something I need to mention before moving on. During my first weeks with the knowledge that I had cancer, it wasn't long before I started reading articles about colon cleansing and liver cleansing/flushing. One habit that I adopted for the first couple of months was to go to sleep each night with a warm water bottle resting against my liver. I actually used one of the modern bottles, now filled with a gel, that can be heated up quickly in the microwave oven. Yes, we have an oven with a microwave function, but this is the only application I use the microwave for.

Why early to bed and early to rise?

I am a morning person by nature, so getting to bed early and rising early probably comes more naturally to me than to other members of my family and friends. This can place a strain on social interaction such as an evening out on the town. And naturally leads to one inevitable question being asked: "Does it really matter how early or late we go to bed, so long as we get a full night's sleep?"

The main reason I opted for the early to bed approach had to do with liver detoxification and body healing, which according to a number of studies I had come across, occurred roughly between 10pm and 2am. It was best to get into the deep REM sleep in that period, which implied going to bed around 9pm - 10pm.

Does winter time or summer time influence these time zones? Do late sunsets or early sunsets influence these time zones? Maybe? Probably? By how much?

Getting to bed late and rising late can disorganize the exile of useless substances (disposing of waste material) from our body. Our ability to sustain exertion is as vital to our health as what we eat and drink.

Getting to bed late and rising early can lead to enduring (chronic) stress, negatively affecting our moods, emotions and abilities to respond quickly, think creatively and feel good about life (vitality).

Do you want to lose some weight?

There exists a relationship between my mealtimes and sleeping schedule that seems to affect my ability to burn off extra fat. For many of us losing weight can be a goal in itself, so you may well be interested in the following "tip" just from that point of view. But for me it was a welcome side-effect, as losing some of my excess body weight would lead to a lesser burden on my liver.

During the first 6 weeks I finished eating for the day with a light dinner some 3 hours before bedtime. This allowed time for relaxation exercises such as yoga 1-2 hours after the meal, just before going to bed. This also allowed at least 11-12 hours between dinner and breakfast: dinner around 6-7pm and breakfast after the morning walk around 7-8am.

For approximately the first 6-8 hours after eating the body is processing the food. The most effective fat burning time seems to be the hours directly after that, say 8-12 hours after eating.

What I have discovered since then, is that if I have a little snack before bedtime, or have the evening meal too late, my body does not seem to switch to a fat burning mode in the early hours of the morning. So that little snack or late meal, however healthy it may have been, becomes an impairment to fat-burning that night.

An understanding of the above mechanism works much better for me, than being presented with blind rules such as "never eat after dinner" or "do not eat large meals" or "chew your food slowly." And a health goal is far more motivational than a "lose weight" goal.

By sticking to rules we may end up doing the same things we do as a result of new insights and understanding. But rules can change, e.g. we jump from one diet to the next. And a diet that is focused on only one aspect, such as losing weight, will throw our bodies out of balance and lead to the derailment of key processes such as fat burning. I blame our modern day body weight yo-yo effect on the introduction of the diet concept. A balanced change in lifestyle, which includes a food plan, can be a change for life. Both a change to save life as well as for the rest of one's life.

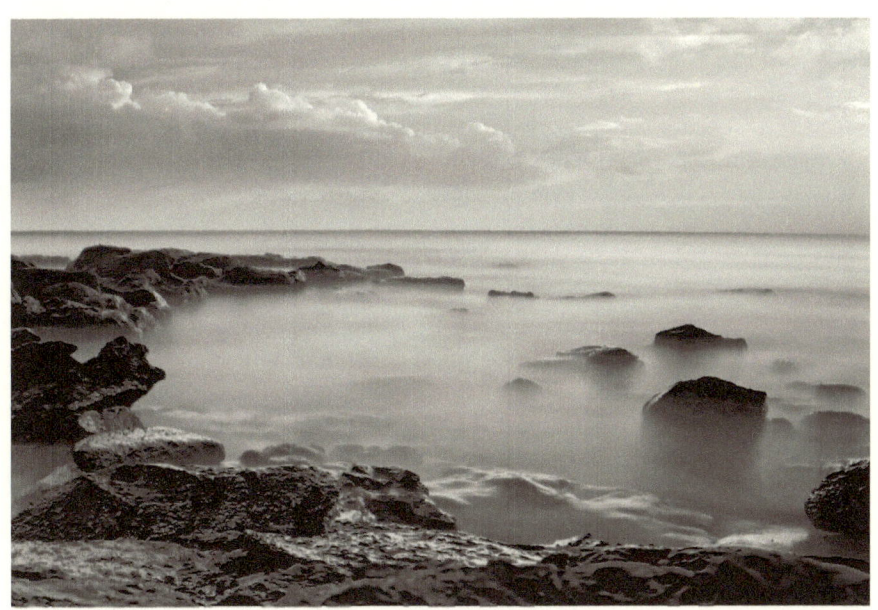

5 DAILY CHALLENGES

One of my biggest challenges continues to be the development and application of a daily routine that fits into my work and social agenda.

Do I prepare my own meals, or does someone else (restaurant/canteen/partner) prepare them for me? Because it is important for me to know what ingredients are going into my meals, and because I enjoy cooking, my decision was to prepare my own meals and meals for my family. And I prefer to invite friends over for a meal instead of the other way around.

Do I do my own shopping? Actually, yes. I try to combine local shopping with my morning walk, and afternoon shopping with a bicycle ride into town.

When can I take breaks to eat, drink, exercise? Each day brings new challenges to interrupt my planned schedule. I am in need of a reference framework to help me plan the day. So I split the day up into four phases, which I explain below. Not only does it help me understand what I am trying to do, but my friends and family now have a better appreciation of my daily routine and why I occasionally make some "inconvenient" decisions. I have lost count of evening meals with friends, originally planned for 6pm that were delayed to after 8pm, that I have skipped because they would otherwise interfere with my schedule.

Can I get to bed by 9pm and asleep by 10pm? Do I want to? As my wife is very much a night person who values a social life, I expected to encounter difficulties getting to sleep by 10pm when she gets to bed around 1am. I also enjoy a good film or television series, and many start around 8:30pm onwards. During the first 6 weeks as a cancer patient it was surprisingly easy to get to sleep by 10pm. Years later this can be a real challenge at times.

Can I make time for an afternoon siesta? Being from Mediterranean origin, the afternoon siesta should be second nature for me. Even Dr. Moerman made a point of emphasizing the importance of an afternoon lie down for cancer patients. And yet, surprising to me, during the first 6 weeks I can only recall making the time for a handful of afternoon siestas!!

Can I enjoy a meal without rushing it? Instead of my afternoon siesta, I have opted for eating and drinking in a relaxed (social) environment... whenever possible. For example, an extended lunch with family and friends.

I split the day up into four phases

For as far as I can recall my favorite number is 4. Just like the four seasons in a year. A rhythmical, phased and enduring cycle. So I attempted to break my daily routine into four logical phases, to help me understand what I am trying to achieve in each phase and how all the phases fit together. Something clear to focus on.

But how to break down the 24 hour cycle into 4 phases? I tried out different approaches, and finally settled for an approach that reminded me of the business life cycle I learned during my younger years as a petroleum engineer in the oil & gas industry, namely:

- exploration
- appraisal

- development & construction
- production & disposal.

Morning 5am - 12am Production & disposal

The focus is on generating output. I do most of my intensive work in the mornings, including exercise and a brisk walk. The morning is when my body disposes of waste material e.g. no. 1 and no. 2 in the toilet, sweat cleanses my pores, a shower washes the skin residues away. My morning walk also helps to clear up my mind and emotional state, when I let all the thoughts and emotions that come to the surface fly away. So as not to interfere with these cleansing processes, I restrict my food and drink consumption to fruits and fruit juices. The juices are combined with a little butter milk (smoothies), and the fruits are combined with a little cottage cheese & flax-seed oil (e.g. the popular Johanna Budwig's Breakfast Recipe to kick off the detoxification process in the morning).

Afternoon 12am - 7pm Exploration

The focus is on processing input. This is the best time to assimilate new information and food. I strive to eat my main meal early afternoon and close with a small meal late afternoon. But more often than not the early afternoon meal comes under time pressure and is kept short and light. Come late afternoon I am faced with the decision to go for a light meal or a large meal. The large meal rules out any light exercise or yoga later in the evening, as my body needs 3-4 hours in-between time. After a light meal 1 hour in-between time is sufficient.

Evening 7pm - 10pm Appraisal

The focus is on reviewing my day. This is the shortest of the four phases, and is a time for (self) reflection, yoga/light exercise at least 1 hour after small meal / 3-4 hours after large meal (it makes sense to take the light meal in the late afternoon, and the larger meal around noon)

Night 10pm - 5am Development & construction

The focus is on general maintenance. My sleep from 10pm - 2am is most important from the point of my body healing itself. During the night my body rebuilds itself. Note: this magical period for healing relates to the daily periods of daylight and nighttime, so it probably makes sense to go to bed a little later in the summer time and a little earlier during the winter months. I wonder what the effects are of living in the Nordic regions where it is nighttime for months on end, and daytime for the rest of the year.

I live each day under a unique set of responsibilities, obligations and priorities that will effect the positioning and duration of each phase within the 24 hour cycle. An awareness of the four phases helps me with my daily decisions of what to do and what not to do at different times of the day.

Maintaining the daily structure

During my first 6 weeks with cancer I had no issues about sticking to my daily structure. But then I started to convince myself that I could ease up here and there. People, places and things started to claim my time and my attention again. *After having started off in a very assertive frame of mind, I found myself sinking back into a more reactive mode.* When I stop being assertive and start reacting more and more to people, places and things, I become more and more irritable. No morning walk because I had gone out with friends to the theater and stayed out late. The piece of cake with coffee to celebrate a friend or family member's birthday. Each of the four phases I had identified for myself presented its own unique challenges, and yet they are all interconnected one-after-the-other into a spiral, steady during the first 6 weeks, but with a clear tendency to spiral downwards under the influence of people, places and things.

Morning: the early morning walk suffers from late nights
Afternoon: the late afternoon meal more often than not slips back into the evening e.g. dinner with friends, back home late from work.
Evening: sitting down in front of the television kills any intended self-reflection or light exercise, as can an evening out with friends. I say can, because a social life with partner and friends can also take place in a quiet atmosphere such as sitting around a camp fire or a terrace overlooking the sea - a time for relaxation, conversation and open reflection.
Night: an evening out, a late night film... people, places and things once again set my bed-time back

I have learned, from trial-and-error, that to regain my structure all I have to do is go on my early morning walk tomorrow morning, and the following morning, and the morning after that, and all the other pieces will gradually fall into place again. This one simple act of assertion is enough to switch off my reactive mode.

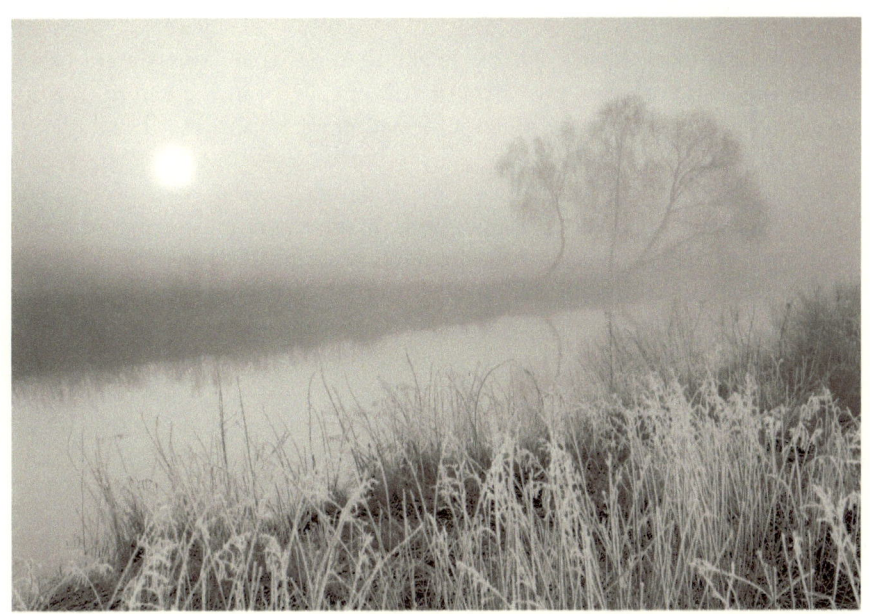

6 HAPPY GOOGLING

I am not going to bore us all here with a list of references and recommended reading, or a summary of all the different cancer treatments and schools of thoughts that exist on cancer and other chronic diseases and health.

And yes, I could write many chapters on all the different avenues that I have explored and still plan to explore.

That's all about my journey.

This book should focus on us, our diverse needs and our personal journeys.

What I do provide, to help us out on our own journeys, is a selection of names, book titles, terms and description phrases that we can google for ourselves – if and when we so desire.

The list is by no means exhaustive and does not cover everything I have come across during the past years or will encounter in the future. But it does serve to illustrate how much information is available that I had never heard of before I had cancer.

On the one hand very enriching, but at the same time very confusing and contradictory, at times mis-informative, covering a whole range of facts and fiction and questionable truths and interpretations, between the extremes of anecdotal stories at one end and science-based evidence at the other.

I have not attempted to order or structure or pre-arrange this list. It's a raw collection of search terms for you, the reader, to browse through and pick and choose from at your discretion.

Happy googling!

OTA Unconventional Cancer Treatments report
Gerson Research Foundation
History of the Gerson therapy
colon cleansing
Bernando Lapallo
Avicenna – The Canon
Hildegard von Bingen – Physica
Greek Arabic medicine
Ayurveda – Unani
Charlotte Gerson - documentary Food Matters
vitamins, minerals, enzymes, phytochemicals, antioxidants
Journal of Clinical Oncology
Dr. Fuhrman – nutritarian
adaptive immune system and an evolutionary older innate immune system
Dr. Robert McCarrison – the medical testament
Murray Grossan, M.D. - Principles of why a placebo works
Burzynski
immunotherapy
human immune system
Danny Hillis: Understanding cancer through proteomics
Carlo Petrini – slow food

innovations in oncology

Wim Hof (the iceman) – breathing technique and visualization

Moerman food plan

qigong

Curcumin Helps Change Gene Function to Combat Cancer

The China Study

EPIC - The European Prospective Investigation into Cancer and Nutrition

The Continuous Update Project (CUP) from the World Cancer Research Fund (WCRF)

prof. dr. Carl Figdor - utilizing the human body's immune system to fight cancer

Clinical trials vs retrospective research

Pharma-Nutrition conference

David Klein Ph.D. - self healing colitis & crohn's

Wim Hof - the yoga practice of Inner Fire, or Tum-mo

Bernie Siegel workshop

neutroponia - neutropenic diet

Dr. David Servan-Schreiber - Anticancer: A New Way of Life

Brandt Grape Cure

Dr. Richard Béliveau and Dr. Denis Gingras - foods that fight cancer

Mediterranean diet

CancerTutor - Cellect-Budwig Protocol

USDA Nutrient Database

Dr. Colin Campbell

Glycemic Index - Glycemic load

slow carbs

chana dal

quinoa - amaranth

goji berries

mung beans

cancer fighting herbs

enzyme-dead foods

enzyme-rich foods - sprouted seeds

gall bladder - olive oil + lemon juice flush

Christopher Hobbs - Natural Liver Therapy

candida and cancer

acid-alkaline balance

Tabata study – tabata training intervals

food synergy

quantum touch - reconnective healing – reiki

Tai Chi and Yoga

mindfulness

biotherapy, immunotherapy, nutritional biotherapy, biological therapy

the living matrix

Danny Dreyer - Chi walking and Chi running

The Leptin Diet: Solving Obesity and Preventing Disease

Qi philosophy - Yin and yang exercises

lymphatic system – exercises

Myofascial release - increasing circulation and lymphatic drainage

Qigong exercises - lymph nodes

Lift Chi Up Pour Chi Down - Zhening, Chi-Lel, Chi Neng

power walking

fox walking – nordic walking – chi walking

Warburg, Gerson, Koch, Moerman

Hans Moolenburgh (in Dutch: u kunt meer dan u denkt – aanvullende maatregelen om kanker te helpen voorkomen en genezen)

Dr Otto Warburg (1883-1970)

Dr Dean Burk (1904-1988)

Dr Max Gerson (1881-1959)

William F. Koch, BA MA Ph.D MD

Dr Cornelis Moerman (1893 - 1988)

Dr. Norman Wardhaugh Walker (January 4, 1886—June 6, 1985)

Vernon Coleman

WCRF - eating well and being active after cancer treatment

Food for the Fight DVD

Dr. Colin Campbell - The China Study

Bernie Siegel, Ian Gawler, Carl Simonton

Henk Fransen - Autobiography of an immune cell

101 Miracles of Natural Healing by Luke Chan

Dr. Linus Pauling (winner of 2 Nobel prizes and founder of orthomolecular medicine)

"The Grape Cure" written by Johanna Brandt (1876-1964)

Dr. Johanna Budwig (1908-2003) - the Budwig diet/flax seed oil

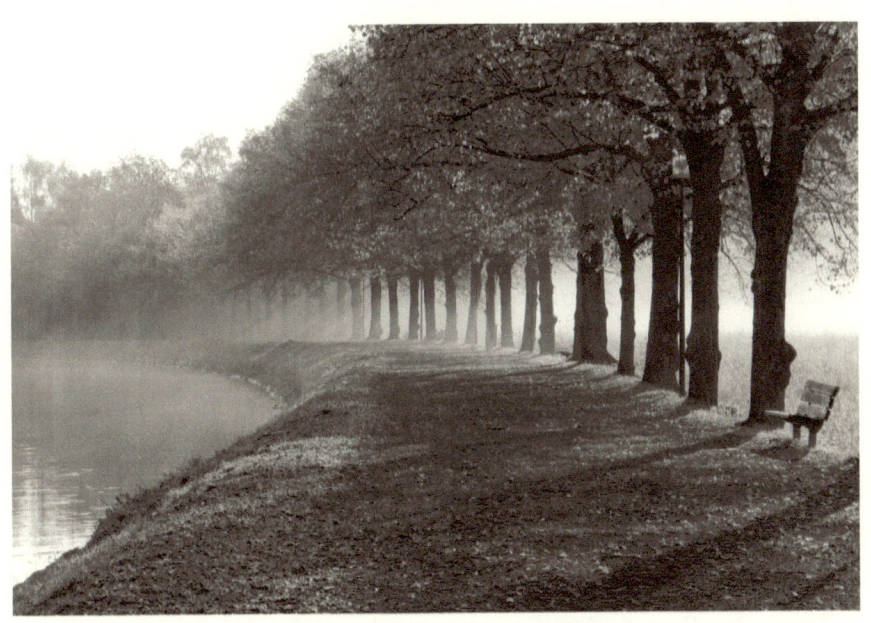

7 EPILOGUE

The liver

This whole book really revolves around the liver and the emphasis placed on taking care of the liver.

There is only one categorical imperative in the fight to survive cancer (this is a different mindset to fighting cancer or a war against cancer), and that is to take care of the liver. There are no minor absolutes.

The lesson of "one categorical imperative" is a lesson I have learned (and forgotten) time and again throughout the course of my life. And it is both as a golfer as well as a cancer patient that I was recently reminded of it (again.)

One of golf's great professional teachers, Ernest Jones (1887–1965), when recalling his first efforts as a teacher, admits that he did not have the slightest idea of how to go about it, he decided to begin a careful study of books on how to teach. He read every book by every leading professional.

He confesses that, with only one exception, the books failed to help him. They merely added to his confusion because of their many contradictions. The exception was a book published in 1887 and entitled "The Art of Golf" by Sir Walter Simpson.

That book started him thinking along a line entirely different from anything he had previously encountered. It emphasized that in golf there is only one categorical imperative, and that is to hit the ball. There are no minor absolutes.

The initial experiences of Ernest Jones, in his search for a way to teach golf, are very similar to my own experiences in my search for a way to control the cancer process. And of all the books that I have studied written by experienced medical professionals, many of which I have found to be inspiring and informative in spite of their many contradictions, it was the title of Dr. Cornelis Moerman's book that pointed me in an entirely different direction than the one proposed by my oncologist.

This book was published in Dutch in 1978 and is entitled "Cancer that results from inadequate nutrition can heal through diet and therapy." I was fortunate to come across this book second-hand just a few days after being told that I had cancer, because it helped me put together a new food plan for myself. This was one of the first steps along the hard path back.

Protective shield

What have I learned about protecting the liver? Three things. Adopt a liver-friendly food plan. Adopt a liver-friendly exercise routine. And adopt a liver-friendly sleep and rest schedule.

And what are the side-effects usually associated with someone who has cancer? Lack of appetite. Lack of energy. The need to rest and to sleep. It's almost as if the cancer process is acting as a protective shield around the liver by cutting out the food processing that is taxing on the liver, preventing the physical and emotional exertions that also tax the liver, and providing the time-out that the liver needs if it is to recuperate.

The cancer process, acting as a protective shield from the attacks of daily life in the surrounding troubled waters, is buying us extra time to perform some life critical repairs.

We decide how to put this extra time to good use.

Modified cancer treatment protocols

Cancer can be many years in the making. Cancer treatments can be many years in their duration. More often than not we discover cancer when our health has hit rock bottom. From this rock bottom we are urged to endure the additional hardships of conventional cancer treatment protocols.

The decision to undergo a cancer treatment is our decision. We, the cancer patients, make the final decision as to which cancer treatment we are going to follow and when.

As much as I would like to see cancer treatment protocols modified to include a 6 week preparation phase, in which the cancer patient is "prepped up" through the liver-friendly life style changes described in this book, reality is that it may still take many more years for the medical establishment to embrace this notion.

But *we* can make *our* own decisions today. I decided not to follow my oncologist's recommendations. This was a risky decision that paid off for me. But I could have decided differently had the conditions been different.

I could have decided to follow one of the cancer treatment protocols suggested by my oncologist, or one suggested during a second or third opinion.

I could have said yes to the cancer treatment, only not now, but in 4-6 weeks time.

I could have then explained what I was going to do in those 6 weeks, and consulted with medical staff as to how my food plan would impact on any hospital stay during the course of the cancer treatment.

I could have requested that a hospital nutritionist be assigned to coach and advise me throughout the duration of the cancer treatment period.

I might have even asked for new scans to be made after the 4-6 weeks preparation and prior to commencing with the cancer treatment, and based on these latest results made a final "Go" or "No Go" decision regarding the proposed cancer treatment.

I personally do not have an issue with surgical removal of these tumors, because this helps with the detoxification of the body, and removes some of the load that our liver has been carrying. But chemo and radiation treatments do not fit into my picture of a body detoxification followed by a rebuilding of our health. The chemo and radiation treatments, by introducing toxic waste into the body, just aggravate the situation for already over-loaded organs, in particular the liver.

So should I ever decide to follow a recommended chemo or radiation therapy, then I will consider delaying this for 4-6 weeks. 4-6 weeks in which I can adopt the lifestyle changes recommended in this book. If after these 4-6 weeks I still decide to go ahead with chemo or radiation therapy, at least I will be in a much healthier state to undergo these therapies. The therapies will also, I believe, be more effective. The unwelcome side-effects from these therapies will be minimized and I will recover faster from these therapies. Add all these aspects up, and a 4-6 week delay will buy me both a better quality of life while undergoing the therapies as well as improve my expected survival rate as a result of the therapies.

And what if my oncologist informs me that my cancer is not nutrition related, but related to a genetic flaw in my constitution? If the flaw is genetic then I would adhere to my lifestyle changes even more rigorously. At the moment I appear to get on well with an 80/20 approach, which is 80% adherence to my preferred lifestyle plan, and a 20% deviation (flexibility) which my family and friends label enjoying life. But if my flaw was genetic, then I would go the whole 100%, as I did during my first few months with cancer.

That's it. I have now said and shared what I wanted to say and share. Preventing and controlling cancer has been as simple as good food, gentle exercise and plenty of sleep. Simple yes, but not always easy.

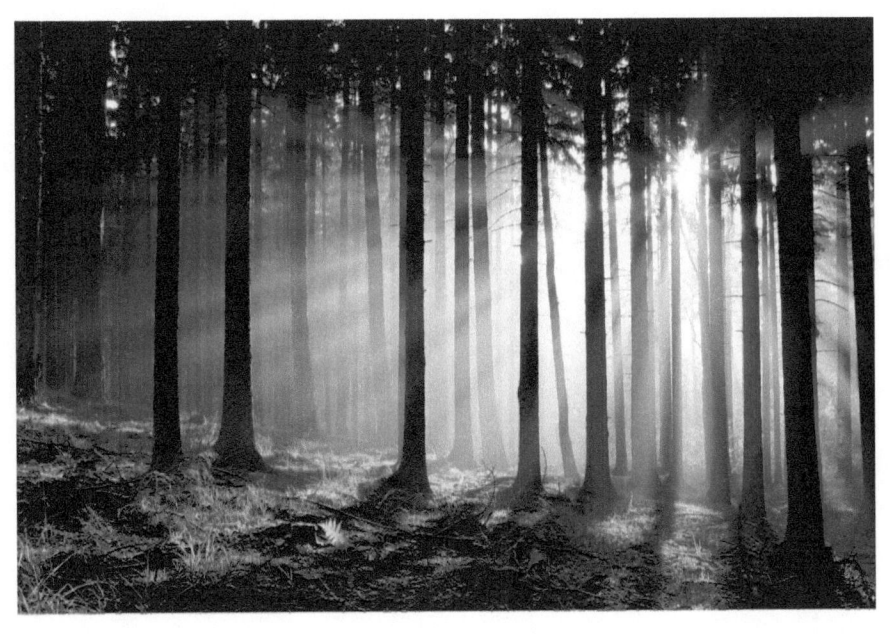

PUBLISHED BY WOLDON PUBLISHING HOUSE 2012

www.ingramcontent.com/pod-product-compliance
Lightning Source LLC
Chambersburg PA
CBHW020402290526
45785CB00005B/2407